# PROS AND CONS OF BEING A VEGETARIAN

## THE ULTIMATE GUIDE

# CYRIL LAKES

# Contents

# CHAPTER ONE

## INTRODUCTION

Giving up on meat, poultry, and seafood is the lifestyle choice of being a vegetarian. Although many people choose to follow a vegetarian diet for moral, environmental, or health-related reasons, there are benefits and drawbacks to this way of eating.

**Advantages:**

Advantages for Your Health: Fruits, vegetables, whole grains, and plant-based proteins are abundant in vitamins, minerals, and antioxidants. A vegetarian diet can also be high in these nutrients. Vegetarian diets may reduce the risk of chronic illnesses like diabetes, heart disease, and some types of cancer, according to research.

Environmental Sustainability: Compared to animal agriculture, the production of plant-based foods often uses less natural resources, such as land and water, and emits less greenhouse gases. Vegetarians can decrease their impact on the environment and support sustainability initiatives by consuming less meat.

Ethical Considerations: Concern for animal welfare and the moral treatment of animals is a common reason for vegetarianism. Steering clear of meat products encourages more humane agricultural methods and lessens the need for animals raised in factories.

Weight management: Compared to omnivorous diets, vegetarian diets often contain fewer calories and saturated fat, which may help with weight loss and maintenance. Foods derived from plants are frequently high in fiber and can support satiety and fullness sensations.

Cooking Diversity and Creativity: Those who follow a vegetarian diet are more inclined to experiment with a greater range of plant-based meals and cooking methods. It can stimulate culinary creativity and result in the discovery of novel tastes, textures, and recipes.

**Cons:**

Potential Nutrient Deficiencies: Vegetarians may be susceptible to inadequacies in protein, iron, zinc, calcium, vitamin B12, and omega-3 fatty acids, among other nutrients. Vegetarians should carefully arrange their diets to make sure they are getting all the nutrients they need from a variety of plant-based sources, supplements, and fortified foods.

Practical and Social Difficulties: Vegetarians may find it more difficult to socialize and eat out, particularly in places where meat is widely consumed. It could take some extra work and compromise to find acceptable vegetarian selections at restaurants or family get-togethers.

Limited Food Options: Vegetarians may need to restrict or cut out specific foods from their diets, depending on their own tastes and nutritional requirements. This might result in a less diversity of food options and possibly monotonous meals.

Possibility of Bad Decisions: Vegetarian cuisine isn't always healthful. Even processed and junk food with vegetarian labels may include high levels of sugar, sodium, and harmful fats. Vegetarians should prioritize whole, minimally processed foods and refrain from consuming an excessive amount of convenience food.

Misconceptions and societal Stigma: Vegetarians may have misconceptions about their dietary choices and societal stigma, such as worries about their protein intake or presumptions about their moral convictions. Dispelling falsehoods and promoting understanding can be achieved by educating others about the advantages and logic of vegetarianism.

There are several possible advantages of vegetarianism for the environment, human health, and animal welfare. But it also poses problems with regard to social dynamics, practical issues, and adequate nutrition. People can adopt a dietary pattern that is in line with their values and objectives by weighing the benefits and drawbacks of vegetarianism and making educated decisions.

## What Vegetarianism Is

One dietary practice known as vegetarianism is the avoidance of meat, poultry, and seafood. For the most part, plant-based meals such fruits, vegetables, grains, legumes, nuts, seeds, and dairy products (for lacto-vegetarians), provide the nutritional requirements of vegetarians. Vegetarianism can be adopted for a variety of reasons, such as cultural, religious, ethical, environmental, or health-related ones. Vegetarianism comes in various forms, such as:

A plant-based diet that eliminates meat, poultry, fish, and eggs but includes dairy products (milk, cheese, and yogurt) is known as lacto-vegetarianism.

Ovo-Vegetarianism: This diet consists of eating eggs while avoiding dairy, beef, poultry, and shellfish.

Meat, poultry, and seafood are not consumed by lacto-ovo vegetarians, who instead consume dairy products and eggs in their diet.

Pescatarianism: This dietary approach excludes meat and poultry but allows fish and seafood in addition to plant-based foods. It is not strictly vegetarian.

Veganism: Vegans follow a plant-based diet in which they abstain from all foods derived from animals, such as dairy, eggs, honey, poultry, and seafood. Beyond dietary restrictions, veganism frequently refers to a way of life that forgoes the use of animals in the production of apparel, cosmetics, and other commercial items.

Many people embrace vegetarianism for a variety of reasons, such as religious or cultural convictions, animal welfare concerns, environmental sustainability, and health promotion. Whatever the particular variant, when carefully thought out and balanced, including a range of plant-based meals to suit nutrient needs, vegetarian diets can offer sufficient nutrition.

## The Origins and Development of Vegetarianism

Vegetarianism has a long history and has evolved as a result of cultural, religious, philosophical, and utilitarian influences spanning thousands of years. Below is a summary of significant turning points and advancements in the history of vegetarianism:

Ancient Civilizations: There is evidence that vegetarian diets were followed in ancient India, Greece, and Egypt, demonstrating the long history of vegetarianism. For thousands of years, Hinduism, Buddhism, and Jainism—among other religious and philosophical traditions—have shaped the practice of vegetarianism in India. Based on moral and physiological concerns, ancient Greek philosophers like Pythagoras and Plato also supported vegetarianism.

Religious and Philosophical Traditions: Vegetarianism is accepted as a moral or spiritual practice in many religious and philosophical traditions. Vegetarianism has become popular among Hindus as a result of the religion's emphasis on ahimsa (non-violence). Similar to this, vegetarianism is supported by Buddhism and Jainism as a way to lessen harm and advance spiritual purity, as well as compassion for all living things.

Europe in the Middle Ages and Renaissance: Vegetarianism saw ups and downs in acceptance throughout Europe during these times. Based on their religious convictions, certain Christian sects, including the Essenes and the Cathars, advocated vegetarianism. Vegetarianism was not, however, universally accepted and was frequently connected to fringe intellectual or religious organizations.

Early Advocacy and Vegetarian Societies: Organized vegetarian movements and advocacy groups began to take shape in Europe and North America during the 18th and 19th centuries. Prominent individuals including Sylvester Graham, William Cowherd, and Thomas Tryon encouraged vegetarianism for moral, ethical, and social grounds. The Vegetarian Society was one of the first groups in the world to encourage and advance vegetarianism; it was established in the United Kingdom in 1847.

Modern Vegetarianism: Throughout the 20th and 21st centuries, vegetarianism has gained global acceptability and popularity. Vegetarianism and veganism are becoming more and more popular due to factors like expanding proof of the health benefits of plant-based diets, animal welfare concerns, and rising environmental awareness.

As the demand for plant-based substitutes grows, vegetarian and vegan menu selections are becoming more readily available in eateries, grocery stores, and food service establishments.

Current Trends and Movements: Vegetarianism and veganism have gained popularity recently as mainstream dietary options that are accepted by individuals of all ages and backgrounds. Plant-based diets have become more commonplace thanks to influencers, athletes, and celebrities, who have also helped normalize and accept them in popular culture. Social media platforms have been crucial in advancing the vegetarian and vegan lifestyles by giving online groups a place to exchange recipes, tools, and encouragement.

# CHAPTER TWO

All things considered, the development and history of vegetarianism show the intricate interaction of practical, ethical, religious, and cultural elements. Although vegetarianism has long been practiced, a number of social, environmental, and health-related factors have led to a considerable increase in the religion's acceptance and popularity in recent years.

## Benefits of a Vegetarian Diet

There are several possible physiological, environmental, and ethical advantages to adopting a vegetarian diet. The following are some advantages of switching to a vegetarian diet:

**Advantages for Health:**

Decreased Risk of Chronic Illnesses: Studies have linked vegetarian diets to a decreased risk of long-term illnesses like obesity, heart disease, high blood pressure, type 2 diabetes, and several types of cancer. Diets based mostly on plants typically have higher levels of fiber, vitamins, minerals, and antioxidants and lower levels of cholesterol and saturated fat, all of which can lead to better health results.

Better Weight control: Because vegetarian diets place a strong emphasis on whole, plant-based meals that are higher in fiber and lower in calories, which promote feelings of fullness and satiety, they may help with weight loss and better weight control.

**Sustainability of the Environment:**

Diminished Carbon Footprint: Diets heavy in plant-based foods have less of an environmental impact than diets heavy in animal products. In general, the production of plant-based foods uses less natural resources such as land and water and emits less greenhouse gases, both of which support environmental sustainability.

Conservation of Resources: Vegetarians contribute to the preservation of resources needed in animal agriculture, including water, land, and energy, by consuming less meat. This can lessen the negative effects of livestock production on the environment, such as habitat degradation, deforestation, and water pollution.

**Moral Aspects to Take into Account:**

Animal Welfare: Concern for the ethical treatment of animals and animal welfare is a common reason for vegetarianism. By abstaining from meat products, you help to promote more compassionate and animal-friendly agricultural methods and lessen the need for animals raised in factories.

Reduction of Animal Suffering: Vegetarians help to lessen animal suffering and foster a more moral and compassionate relationship with animals by giving up meat consumption.

Preservation of ecosystems: By lowering the demand for land used for cattle grazing and feed production, plant-based diets contribute to the preservation of natural ecosystems and biodiversity. Ecological balance and biodiversity can only be preserved by safeguarding ecosystems and wildlife habitats.

**Various and Healthful Food Selections:**

Variety of Plant-Based Foods: Fruits, vegetables, whole grains, legumes, nuts, seeds, and plant-based proteins are just a few of the plant-based foods that vegetarian diets promote. This type offers a broad range of vitamins, minerals, and nutrients that are essential for good health and wellbeing.

Experimentation with Novel Flavors and Recipes: Changing to a vegetarian diet can stimulate culinary innovation and result in the creation of novel flavors, textures, and recipes. Trying out different plant-based products can broaden one's culinary horizons and foster a deeper respect for plant-based diets.

All things considered, there are a lot of potential health, ethical, and environmental advantages to being a vegetarian. People can improve their own health and contribute to a more just, sustainable, and compassionate food system by switching to a plant-based diet.

A vegetarian diet has numerous advantages, but there are also some possible disadvantages or difficulties to take into account. The following are some drawbacks of vegetarianism:

**Possible inadequacies in nutrients:**

Some nutrient shortages, including as those in vitamin B12, iron, zinc, calcium, omega-3 fatty acids, and protein, may be present in vegetarians. When compared to animal-derived sources, plant-based sources of certain nutrients may be less accessible or present in smaller quantities, necessitating careful planning and supplementation to guarantee adequate intake.

**Few Food Options:**

Vegetarians may need to limit or cut out specific foods from their diets, depending on their own preferences and nutritional requirements. This might result in a less selection of foods and possibly monotonous meals. In certain contexts, it can be difficult to find appropriate vegetarian options when dining out or socializing.

**Practical and Social Difficulties:**

Vegetarians may find it more difficult to socialize and eat out, particularly in places where meat is often consumed. It could take more work and compromise to find acceptable vegetarian options at dining establishments, get-togethers with family, or social functions. Some people could also experience peer or family pressure or criticism for the food choices they make.

**Possibility of Making Bad Decisions:**

Not every vegetarian cuisine is healthful by nature. Even processed and junk food items with vegetarian labels may include high levels of added sugars, salts, harmful fats, and chemicals. Vegetarians run the risk of becoming overly dependent on processed meat substitutes or convenience foods, which can lead to poor nutritional quality and detrimental health effects.

**Misconceptions and Social Stigma:**

Vegetarians may experience prejudice from the community or misunderstandings about their dietary choices, such as preconceived notions about their morality or worries about their protein intake. There may be unfavorable preconceptions or misconceptions regarding vegetarianism held by some individuals, which can cause misinterpretations or prejudices against vegetarians.

**Possibility of Insufficient Protein Consumption:**

Since protein is a necessary component for good health, vegetarians must make sure they consume adequate protein from plant-based sources. Although there is protein in many plant meals, some may not be as complete as animal sources or may even have less protein overall. To satisfy their demands for protein, vegetarians may need to eat a range of foods high in protein.

# CHAPTER THREE

**Having Trouble Locating Vegetarian-Friendly Choices:**

Vegetarians may find it difficult to locate appropriate dietary options in specific areas or cultural contexts where vegetarian-friendly options may be few or less easily accessible. When traveling or residing in places with limited access to fresh vegetables or vegetarian-friendly dining establishments, this can be very troublesome.

Vegetarians must be aware of these possible difficulties and take proactive measures to overcome them, such as thoughtful meal planning, supplements when necessary, and public support of their dietary choices. Many of these disadvantages can be successfully avoided with careful preparation and knowledge, enabling people to reap the rewards of a vegetarian diet while minimizing any possible negative effects.

## Resolving and Reducing the Drawbacks

It takes proactive measures and thoughtful approaches to address and mitigate the possible disadvantages or difficulties of being a vegetarian in order to guarantee a healthy and fulfilling diet. The following are some strategies to address and lessen the drawbacks of being a vegetarian:

**Resolving Nutritional Inadequacies:**

Become Informed: Find out which nutrients, such as protein, iron, zinc, calcium, vitamin B12, and omega-3 fatty acids, may be deficient in a vegetarian diet. Deficiencies can be avoided by being aware of which foods have these nutrients and how to best absorb them.

Plan Balanced Meals: If you're a lacto-vegetarian, make sure your diet includes a range of nutrient-rich foods, such as fruits, vegetables, whole grains, legumes, nuts, and seeds, as well as plant-based protein sources. To guarantee sufficient nutritional intake, create balanced meals that incorporate a variety of these food categories.

Take Supplementation Into Consideration: To address specific nutrient deficiencies, take supplements into consideration based on individual needs and dietary habits. Seek advice from a qualified nutritionist or healthcare provider to ascertain whether supplements is appropriate and essential for you.

**Increasing the Variety of Food Options:**

Try New Foods: To broaden your gastronomic horizons and avoid food boredom, delve into an extensive array of plant-based meals and components. To keep things interesting, experiment with different fruits, vegetables, grains, legumes, herbs, spices, and plant-based protein sources in your meals.

Get Creative in the Kitchen: Try out new tastes, cooking methods, and recipe ideas to add excitement and enjoyment to vegetarian meals. Cookbooks, the internet, cooking schools, and vegetarian-friendly dining establishments are good places to look for ideas.

Look for Vegetarian-Friendly Options: Do some research and determine whether local eateries, cafes, and restaurants are vegetarian-friendly. Nowadays, a lot of restaurants include vegetarian menu selections or may fulfill particular dietary demands if they are informed in advance. Never be afraid to ask for vegetarian options or to have existing menu items modified when you're dining out.

**Overcoming Practical and Social Obstacles:**

Communicate Your Needs: Be honest and forthright with friends, family, and coworkers regarding your dietary requirements and preferences. Inform them ahead of time about your vegetarian diet so they can make arrangements for dinners or get-togethers that suit your needs.

Bring Your Own meal: If there aren't many vegetarian alternatives available at an event or gathering, think about bringing a meal to share with other attendees. This not only introduces others to wonderful vegetarian cuisine, but it also guarantees that you'll have something to eat that fits your dietary choices.

Be Adaptable and Flexible: Acknowledge that not every circumstance will accommodate your dietary requirements, and be ready to adjust and become flexible as needed. Without feeling constrained or cheated, concentrate on choosing the best course of action for you in each particular circumstance.

**Making Sure You're Eating Enough Protein:**

Include Foods High in Protein: When planning your meals, try to include a range of plant-based protein sources, such as quinoa, almonds, seeds, chickpeas, tofu, tempeh, edamame, and seitan. For the purpose of promoting muscular health, satiety, and general nutrient balance, try to include protein with every meal.

Mix Complementary Proteins: Include complementary protein sources in your meals, such as beans and rice, hummus and whole grain pita, or tofu and quinoa, to make sure your body is getting all the important amino acids it needs. This contributes to the creation of complete protein sources that contain every necessary amino acid.

Through the application of these tactics, vegetarians can proficiently tackle and alleviate any potential obstacles linked to their dietary preferences, guaranteeing a wholesome, nourishing, and gratifying diet that promotes the highest possible level of health and well-being.

## Summary

Insights into the advantages, difficulties, and experiences of vegetarianism can be gained from the personal reflections and testimonies of those who have followed this lifestyle. Here are some vegetarians' testimonies and personal reflections:

**Advantages for Health:**

"Since transitioning to a vegetarian diet, I've noticed significant improvements in my overall health. I have more energy, my digestion has improved, and I've lost weight without feeling deprived. Plus, knowing that I'm nourishing my body with wholesome, plant-based foods gives me a sense of vitality and well-being." - Sarah says,

**Moral Aspects to Take into Account:**

"Becoming a vegetarian was one of the best decisions I've ever made for both my health and my conscience. I simply couldn't reconcile my love for animals with the idea of supporting industries that exploit and mistreat them. Choosing a vegetarian lifestyle allows me to align my values with my actions and live more authentically." - Alexandra

**Effect on the Environment:**

"As an environmentalist, adopting a vegetarian diet was a no-brainer for me. I wanted to reduce my carbon footprint and minimize my impact on the planet, so cutting out meat was a logical step. Knowing that I'm contributing to environmental sustainability every time I sit down to eat brings me a sense of fulfillment and purpose." - Maya says,

**Social Difficulties:**

"While I'm committed to my vegetarian lifestyle, there have been times when it's been challenging, especially in social situations. I've had to navigate awkward conversations, endure skeptical looks, and politely decline offers of meat-based dishes. However, the support of like-minded friends and the satisfaction of staying true to my beliefs make it all worthwhile." - Jason says,

**Investigating Cuisine:**

"Transitioning to a vegetarian diet has opened up a whole new world of culinary possibilities for me. I've discovered a wealth of delicious and nutritious plant-based recipes that I never would have tried otherwise. Cooking and experimenting with vegetarian ingredients has become a creative and enjoyable adventure that brings me joy every day." - Emily said,

**Physical Capabilities:**

"As an athlete, I was initially concerned that switching to a vegetarian diet would compromise my performance and recovery. However, I've found that with careful planning and attention to my nutritional needs, I'm able to fuel my body effectively and maintain peak performance on a plant-based diet. In fact, I've never felt better or stronger!" - David says,

These testimonies and introspective thoughts highlight the variety of reasons, encounters, and advantages connected to vegetarianism. Even though every person's experience is different, these tales demonstrate the advantages of leading a vegetarian diet in terms of ethics, the environment, health, and personal fulfillment.

**THE END**

www.ingramcontent.com/pod-product-compliance
Lightning Source LLC
Chambersburg PA
CBHW051926250726

48659CB00002B/855